Guidelines GP Referrals in Dermatology

Robin Russell-Jones FRCP

Secretary, London Dermatology Planning Group

I n 1998 Schering-Plough will be celebrating its 50th anniversary in the research and manufacture of dermatological products. In commemoration of this occasion, Schering-Plough is distributing this book to physicians as part of its continuing professional education service program to dermatology.

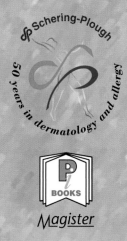

Magister

ACKNOWLEDGEMENTS

M any thanks to the photographic department at St John's Institute of Dermatology for providing the clinical photographs for this publication.

A note about the author

Dr Russell-Jones FRCP, is a Consultant Dermatologist at Ealing Hospital and Hammersmith Hospital, London. He is Director of the Skin Tumour Unit at St John's Institute of Dermatology, London, and Secretary of the London Dermatology Planning Group.

First published by Publishing Initiatives (Europe) Ltd (Magister) in Great Britain 1997

ISBN 1 873839 42 1

Printed and bound in Great Britain by Printarea Ltd, Units 4 & 5 Newgate Lane, Fareham, Hampshire PO14 1BP.

Further copies of *Guidelines for GP referrals in dermatology* may be obtained from Pi Books, a division of Magister. This publication reflects the views and experience of the author and not necessarily those of Magister

Any product mentioned in this book should be used in accordance with the prescribing information prepared by the manufacturer. Neither the author nor the publisher can accept responsibility for any detrimental consequences arising from the information contained herein. Dosages given are for guidance purposes only. No sanctions or endorsements are made for any drug or compound at present under clinical investigation.

CONTENTS

CONTENTS

A recent audit of London GPs showed that 92% of respondents wanted guidelines for dermatology patients in primary care.

The purpose of these guidelines is to outline basic management strategies for common skin disorders and to identify those patients who require referral to hospital. They have been drawn up by the London Dermatology Planning Group (LDPG) in conjunction with GP colleagues and patient groups. Our particular thanks are due to Dr Andrew Warin, Consultant Dermatologist in Exeter, who has produced similar guidelines previously.

It is hoped that GPs will use these guidelines and find them helpful in their day-to-day work. Feedback would be most welcome, as it is intended to produce revised editions in the future.

Before producing these guidelines a survey was conducted of approximately 700 new GP referrals to a London DGH. This revealed that 68% of skin referrals required hospital-based facilities, either for diagnosis (31%) or for treatment (37%).

Twenty-one per cent of referrals were once-only visits (Category 2). No specialised procedures were required, and patients were sent back to the referring GP either with a definite diagnosis (Category 2A) or with advice on management (Category 2B).

A further 11% of patients were referred for minor surgical procedures, such as curettage, shave biopsy or cryotherapy (Category 3). Although these referrals could be managed in the community, it assumes that GPs are given sufficient time and incentive to undertake such procedures and are provided with the necessary equipment and training.

These guidelines are concerned mainly with treatment and should reduce the number of patients in Category 2B, and encourage GPs to obtain the facilities necessary for patients in Category 3. However, there is also potential for reducing the number of patients in Category 2A. Pigmented lesions in particular cause diagnostic difficulties and considerable patient anxiety. It is worth remembering that if a mole can be covered by the blunt end of a pencil, then melanoma is an unlikely diagnosis. Equally, melanoma is exceedingly rare in children.

Table 1 summarises the results of this survey.

Table 1

Analysis of GP referrals
Category 1: 68%

Hospital-based facilities needed
  A For diagnosis (31%)
  B For treatment (38%)

Category 2: 21%
Hospital-based facilities not needed   Advice on diagnosis (2A) or management (2B)
Category 3: 11%
Minor surgical procedures

ACNE

A cne is a source of many referrals to hospital. In theory, patients only require referral if they need investigations to exclude virilising causes of acne (e.g. polycystic ovaries) or if treatment with *Roaccutane*, which is a hospital-only drug, is contemplated. Occasionally, a course of ultraviolet B is used in patients who cannot use other types of treatment, e.g. pregnant women.

Topical treatment

Mild cases of acne can be managed with topical preparations only. All patients should be tried on benzoyl peroxide; concentrations vary from 2.5% to 10%. Start with the weaker preparation and move on to the stronger one after two weeks, if tolerated. If several strengths are prescribed on the same prescription then there is only one prescription charge to the patient.

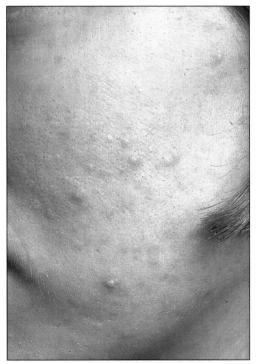

Figure 1 - Mild facial acne showing closed comedones and pustule formation.

Benzoyl peroxide should be applied once or twice daily. It may irritate the skin but this usually settles with continued use. Genuine allergy to benzoyl peroxide is rare. It is a bleach, so care should be taken with towels and bedding.

If benzoyl peroxide is ineffective or poorly tolerated, topical antibiotics are an alternative. These are applied twice daily and include clindamycin (*Dalacin T*), tetracycline (*Topicycline*) and erythromycin (*Stiemycin* or *Zineryt*).

Retin-A is an effective keratolytic, particularly useful in comedonal acne. It is available as *Retin-A* cream at 0.025% and 0.05%, and as

Retin-A gel at 0.01% and 0.025%. It tends to irritate and produce erythema but this usually improves with use, so start with the lower concentration once daily and build up to the stronger concentration twice daily, if the patient will tolerate this.

Isotrex gel has a similar action to *Retin-A*, though it is somewhat less irritant. It is the topical form of *Roaccutane* and may also benefit acne by reducing sebum secretion. Neither *Retin-A* nor *Isotrex* gel should be used in pregnancy.

Oral antibiotic therapy

If a patient requires antibiotics orally then start with oxytetracycline 500 mg bd one hour before meals or four hours after a meal. Keep the patient on this dose for **six months at least**. Do not be concerned if a patient requires oxytetracycline for a year or longer. Patients are still sent to the clinic stating that they have failed to respond to oxytetracycline, even though they have only been taking it for four to six weeks.

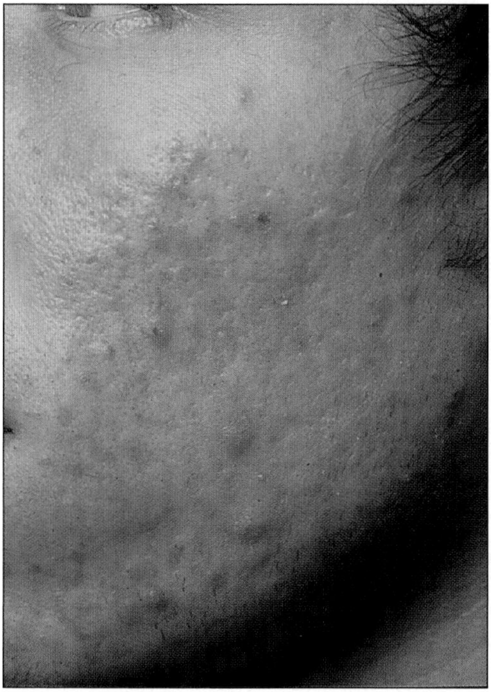

Oxytetracycline is a well-tolerated drug but should not be given to children or pregnant women. There have been occasional reports of benign intracranial hypertension with long-term use of tetracyclines, so persistent headaches should be taken seriously in this group of patients.

Alternative antibiotics include doxycycline (e.g. *Vibramycin* 100 mg daily) or minocycline (*Minocin MR* 100 mg daily). These tetracyclines are better absorbed but with *Minocin* there is a risk of bluish pigmentation

Figure 2 - Moderately severe facial acne showing inflammatory papules/small nodules and scarring.

of the skin with long-term use. This can be long-lasting or even permanent. If patients do not tolerate tetracyclines, then erythromycin 500 mg bd is an alternative. All antibiotics need to be prescribed for six months to obtain maximum benefit.

Acne and the pill

Female patients on a combined oral contraceptive pill who are prescribed antibiotics for their acne need to take additional contraceptive measures, at least for the first month.

Progestogen-only pills and some combined contraceptive pills are liable to aggravate acne. Female patients with acne can be prescribed *Dianette*; this contains 35 µg of ethinyloestradiol (which is beneficial to acne) combined with 2 mg of cyproterone acetate, which is an anti-androgen. It is an effective oral contraceptive, provided it is taken regularly and can be used as a treatment for acne, even in female patients not requiring contraception.

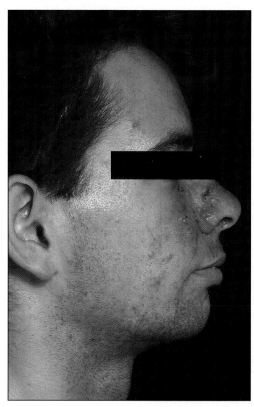

The above treatments can, of course, be used in combination. An oral antibiotic can be combined with benzoyl peroxide or *Isotrex*; *Dianette* can be combined with a topical antibiotic, etc. Only if patients have failed to respond to the above treatments should they be referred to hospital.

It is important to recognise that none of these treatments represents a cure for acne. They are designed to control the condition for as

Figure 3 - Severe facial acne showing nodule and cyst formation before treatment with *Roaccutane*.

long as it is active, and thus reduce any long-term cosmetic problems such as pigmentation or scarring.

When to refer a patient with acne

- Patients who are unresponsive to conventional therapy or whose acne recurs after adequate courses of antibiotics.

- Patients in whom acne is causing unacceptable cosmetic problems: particularly female patients with dark skin which pigments easily.

- Female patients who have evidence of virilisation, that is hirsuties, irregular periods, infertility or late-onset acne, may need investigation to exclude an underlying endocrinological cause. However, unless acne is the presenting symptom, it is probably more appropriate to refer such patients to an endocrinology clinic.

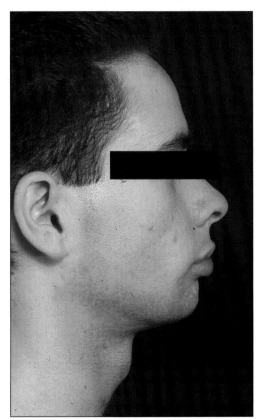

Figure 4 - Same patient as in Figure 3 after treatment with *Roaccutane*.

Oral retinoids

Patients with nodular cystic acne often respond poorly to the therapies outlined and require treatment with oral retinoids. 13-cis retinoic acid (*Roaccutane*) is a dramatically effective drug which will not only clear severe cases of acne but often prevents recurrence in the future. The treatment is given for 16 weeks at a dosage of up to 1 mg/kg; patients are warned about the likely side-effects, particularly cheilitis. Fasting lipids and liver function tests are monitored during therapy

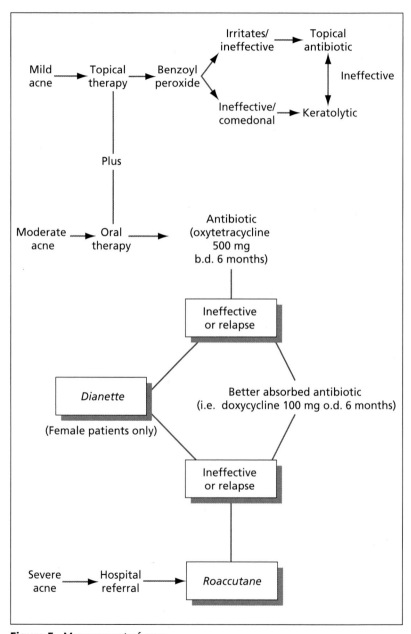

Figure 5 - Management of acne.

and, since the drug is teratogenic, it is absolutely crucial that women do not become pregnant either during treatment or for at least one month after treatment is discontinued. Some patients require a second course of *Roaccutane* (approximately 10%) but recurrences are seldom as severe as at presentation.

ECZEMA/
DERMATITIS

Eczema is a source of many referrals to hospital, particularly in children. Approximately 15% of children develop eczema in the first five years of life and the vast majority of these can be managed in the GP surgery.

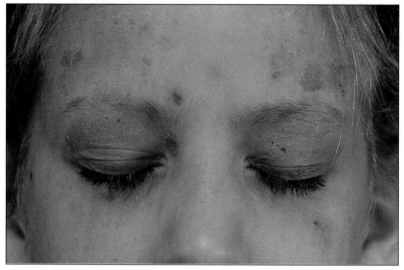

Figure 6 - Atopic eczema in childhood with involvement of the upper eyelids and secondary excoriation.

Patients with eczema may need referral:

- If their eczema is resistant to conventional therapy.

- In order to exclude alternative diagnoses (such as fungal infection or scabies) or

- because the eczema has become secondarily infected, either with a staphylococcal folliculitis or eczema herpeticum.

- If immunosuppressive therapy with azathioprine or cyclosporin is contemplated.

- For exclusion of allergic contact dermatitis. This is a type-IV delayed hypersensitivity reaction to contact allergens such as nickel, rubber, leather, cosmetics, medicaments and other substances which may come in contact with the skin.

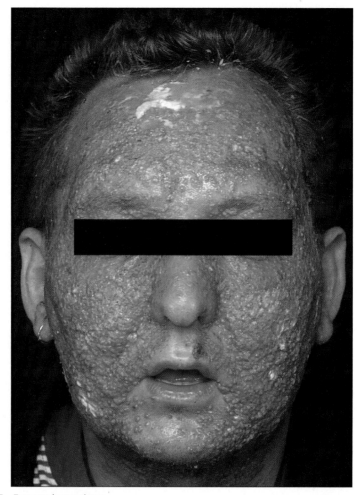

Figure 7 - Eczema herpeticum.

Patch tests

The diagnostic procedure for establishing the presence of allergic contact dermatitis is to carry out patch tests, which take five days to complete. On day 1 (Monday) the patient attends the outpatient department and has the Standard European Battery (the 30 commonest allergens) applied to his/her back, together with any other substances to which the patient or doctor thinks s/he might be allergic. The

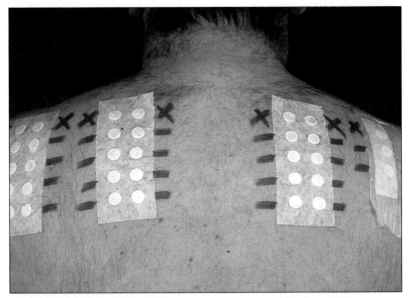

Figure 8 - Patch tests applied to upper back (standard European battery).

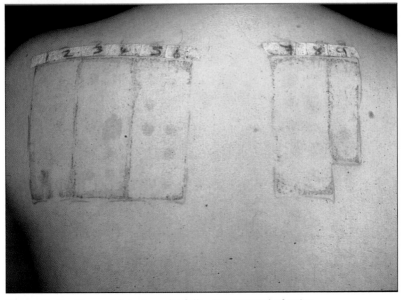

Figure 9 - Positive patch test results following removal of strips.

patient returns two days later (Wednesday) to have the patch test removed and a first reading carried out; and again on Friday for a second patch test reading to be carried out.

Many children with eczema are sent for 'allergy testing'. In fact, patch testing is seldom needed in children with a constitutional (usually atopic) pattern of eczema. Prick testing may be carried out in these children but this is only relevant to the investigation of asthma or hay fever, with which their eczema may be associated. Prick testing does not help in the management of atopic eczema. It is therefore misleading to inform parents that a child with atopic eczema is being referred to the hospital for allergy testing.

The following patterns of eczema should raise your suspicions of an allergic contact dermatitis, where patch testing may be useful:

1. Eyelid, face or perioral eczema as an isolated feature (these sites may, of course, be involved in atopic eczema or seborrhoeic eczema).

2. Otitis externa.

3. Either hand dermatitis or foot dermatitis. Allergic contact dermatitis tends to be worse on the dorsum of the hands or feet, whereas endogenous patterns tend to affect the palms and soles.

4. Eczema associated with venous ulcers.

5. Unusual patterns of eczema, particularly asymmetrical patterns.

6. Finally, if a patient with longstanding endogenous eczema suddenly deteriorates, consider allergy to the medicaments s/he is using. Patients can become allergic to virtually any topically-applied substance, even topical steroids, and this can only be established by appropriate patch tests.

7. Contact allergic dermatitis is, of course, very common in occupationally-exposed groups, e.g. dentists, hairdressers, printers, etc. Any suspicion of an occupationally-related dermatitis merits referral to hospital.

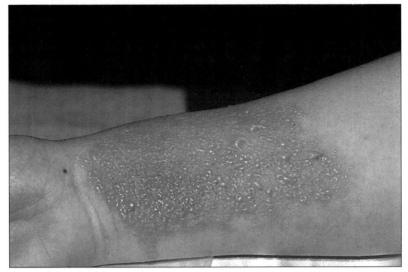

Figure 10 - Allergic contact dermatitis on wrist from application of perfume.

Management of eczema in children

Children with eczema do have sensitive skin. This means that it is easily irritated by non-specific irritants, such as soaps, detergents, washing-up liquid, bubble baths and, sometimes, wool. Such substances should be avoided in children with active eczema. Emollients, such as *Emulsiderm, Oilatum emollient, Balneum bath oil*, etc., should be used for bathing. Aqueous cream or emulsifying ointment should be used instead of soap. For washing-up, rubber gloves with cotton linings should be worn, biological detergents should be avoided and clothes should be well rinsed. Wool next to the skin should be avoided. Cotton is probably better than synthetic fibres.

Children with eczema also have dry skin and dryness can lead to itching. This can be corrected by regular use of moisturising creams such as *Unguentum Merck, E45 Cream, Diprobase*, etc. Adequate supplies should be made available (up to 250 g weekly).

Children will vary as to which moisturiser suits them best so it is worth trying out several different creams. Very dry skin can be treated with *Calmurid* or 50/50 mixture (which contains equal parts of white soft paraffin and liquid paraffin).

There is no reason why children cannot keep a supply of moisturising creams at school, if they need treatment during the day. The regular use of soap substitutes and moisturisers is often all the treatment necessary to control mild cases of eczema in children.

Involving the practice nurse in the management of eczema is very helpful for some children, particularly if medicated bandages are used in treatment.

Steroid treatment

A. Children Active eczema presents as inflamed skin which is red, itchy and scaly. Acute eczema may present with blistering and weeping, but this is uncommon in children with atopic eczema. Active eczema requires treatment with an anti-inflammatory agent. Ointments containing tar have been used in the past but they are messy, irritant and poorly tolerated by most eczema sufferers. For many years steroid creams and ointments have been the mainstay of treatment. Ointments are better for children with dry skin but creams are more cosmetically acceptable. They are usually applied once or twice daily and are probably most effective when used after a bath, when the skin is well hydrated.

Because treatment may need to be continued on a long-term basis, it is important to use the weakest steroid that will effectively control the skin condition. Steroids are divided into four grades:

1. Mild   2. Moderate

3. Potent   4. Very potent.

Most children with eczema can be managed with once- or twice-daily applications of a mild topical steroid, such as 1% hydrocortisone ointment. Moderately strong steroids, such as *Eumovate* or 1:4 *Betnovate* can be used for resistant areas of eczema or in the event of flare-ups. Potent steroids, such as full-strength *Betnovate*, *Propaderm*, *Metosyn*, *Synalar*, etc., are very rarely necessary in children and should not be used on the face. Potent steroids may suppress the pituitary-adrenal axis, particularly if used over large areas of skin or over long periods of time.

Some potent topical steroids, for example *Elocon* and *Cutivate*, are metabolised more quickly than conventional steroids and carry less risk of pituitary-adrenal suppression. However, there is no evidence that local effects on the skin, such as atrophy or telangiectasia, are diminished compared with other topical steroids.

B. Adults Adult patients with eczema may need to use potent steroids in the following clinical situations:

- Areas that are resistant to moderately potent steroids, e.g. areas of chronic lichenification.

- Active areas of eczema that are of limited extent, e.g. discoid eczema.

- Eczema affecting the palms and soles where the skin is thicker and potent steroids may need to be applied under occlusion.

Problems with eczema management and some referrals to hospital could be avoided if acute exacerbations of eczema are dealt with by a short course of potent topical steroids.

Again, the same general principles apply, that the potent steroids should be used for a limited period of time, usually two to three weeks, in order to bring the condition under control before changing to a less potent steroid. Secondly, areas such as the face and flexural areas should be avoided wherever possible.

Eczema and diet

The role of diet in eczema is by no means clear but it has been suggested that certain foods may provoke or exacerbate eczema. It has also been shown that some children, but by no means all, improve if they are put onto diets which are free from eggs, cow's milk and other dairy products. The most certain way of testing whether a child is sensitive to certain foods is to eliminate those substances from the diet and to observe the child, to see whether the eczema improves. If there is no improvement after one month then there is no purpose in continuing with the diet. If, however, the eczema does improve then the next stage is to re-administer the food to see if this is followed by a deterioration in the skin. Ideally, this should be done in co-operation with the dietitian, particularly in the case of young children, who may require milk substitutes such as soya milk.

Even if parents are convinced that a child's skin deteriorates with a particular food, this may not last throughout childhood. Remember, it is not easy for children to adhere strictly to a diet, particularly once

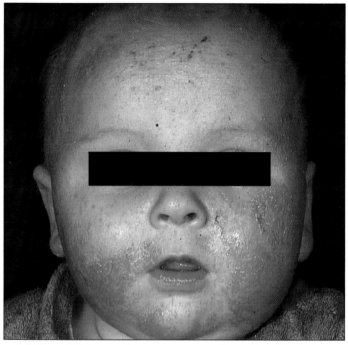

Figure 11 - Infantile eczema affecting the face with evidence of secondary bacterial infection.

they start going to school. It is also not a good idea to change a child's diet repeatedly in the belief that there must be some dietary factor responsible for his or her eczema.

It is important to realise that dietary manipulation (either withdrawal or challenge) is the only reliable method of establishing the role of diet in atopic eczema. Prick tests or blood tests are unreliable and have little or no part to play in the investigation or management of children with atopic eczema.

Acute flare-up of eczema

Eczema may flare spontaneously, without any precipitating cause. This can usually be managed by increasing the potency of the topical steroid and/or prescribing an antihistamine. Some children find that their eczema is worse in the summer (where drying or overheating may have an effect); others find it is worse in the winter, where cold has a deleterious effect. If a child's eczema deteriorates suddenly then swabs should be taken to exclude secondary bacterial infection. *Staphylococcus aureus* is the organism usually responsible and appropriate therapy with erythromycin or flucloxacillin is effective. Repeated bacterial infections or colonisation of eczema by herpes simplex (eczema herpeticum) requires referral to hospital. In older children and, more particularly, in adults, consider the possibility of contact sensitivity to topically-applied medicaments.

Psychological factors are often said to play a large part in eczema. However, it is probably untrue and unfair to state that eczema is the result of stress, since the implication of this is that if only the patient could 'get a grip' psychologically, then their eczema would disappear. If there is a relationship between eczema and stress, it works both ways since bad eczema is a source of severe stress for patients, both in their domestic life and at school. It is also true to say that if a patient is under stress s/he may tend to scratch more and this can aggravate eczema, either through lichenification or through secondary infection. This may go some way to explaining why children with eczema so commonly improve when they go on holiday during the summer.

What of the future?

It is important to explain to parents that the tendency to develop eczema is inherited and is closely associated with other inherited conditions, such as asthma or hay fever (the atopic syndrome). It follows, therefore, that the purpose of treatment is to control rather than cure the condition, so that the child's discomfort is minimised and the child can lead a normal, active life until such time as the condition remits spontaneously.

It is also true that the prevalence of eczema is increasing (as are other atopic disorders). Family size is a possible explanation. It is known, for example, that a first-born child is three times more likely to develop hay fever than is a fifth-born child.

The vast majority of children with eczema improve spontaneously with age and relatively few still have eczema when they are teenagers. However, the tendency to develop eczema does not disappear completely and it is not uncommon for eczema to flare up during adult life, if an unsuitable occupation is chosen. Thus, hairdressers or garage mechanics commonly develop hand eczema when their skin is exposed continuously to shampoos, oils or detergents. Similarly, most hospitals will not accept nurses for training if they have active eczema. If a child has eczema and is thinking of a manual career, it is probably worth discussing this with the patient and parents, before they reach a final decision.

Finally, it is important to remember that children often need support in coping with eczema. Patience and the encouragement of a regular treatment routine are among the most important aspects of management. Patients who wish to learn more about eczema can contact:

The National Eczema Society
163 Eversholt Street, London NW1 113U, Tel: 0171-388 4097

Table 3 **Management of eczema**

Mild eczema	• Avoid irritants (i.e. strong soaps, detergent, bubble baths) • Bath oil • Moisturisers (after bathing) • Mild topical steroid if necessary (i.e. 1% hydrocortisone ointment)
Moderate eczema	As above plus: • Soap substitutes • Regular topical steroid (e.g. 1% hydrocortisone ung.) • Combine with topical antibiotic if infected (e.g. *Fucidin H*, *Vioform HC*, etc.) • Moderately potent topical steroid if necessary • Nocturnal antihistamine • Dietary intervention
Severe eczema	As above plus: • Potent topical steroid if necessary • Occlusive bandaging • Oral antibiotics if clinically indicated • Regular antihistamines
Refer to hospital for	• Repeated infections • Consideration of immunosuppressive therapy • Patch testing

FUNGAL INFECTION

There are three principal classes of fungi which cause superficial infections of the skin.

Tinea

Tinea, i.e. dermatophyte infections or ringworm, are keratinophilic fungi which can affect hair, skin and nails. It is the only fungus for which griseofulvin is effective and also represents the main indication for terbinafine orally (*Lamisil*); 80% of nail infections are cleared by three months of *Lamisil* but remember it takes a year for the nail to grow out normally.

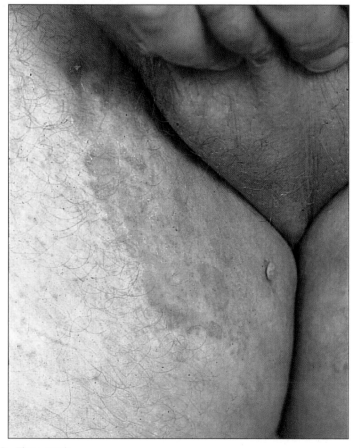

Figure 12 - Tinea cruris.

Pityriasis versicolor

This is due to a yeast-type fungus known as *Malassezia furfur*. Spores are present on all human skin but the spores proliferate to form hyphae and produce a rash in those patients who provide a suitable environment. The aim of treatment is, therefore, not to eradicate the infection completely but to limit the spore population. The simplest treatment is to apply a fungicidal lotion such as *Nizoral* shampoo or *Selsun* shampoo (which contains selenium sulphide) and wash off after half an hour. If this is done daily for a week and then once a week or once a fortnight thereafter, it will prevent recurrence of the condition.

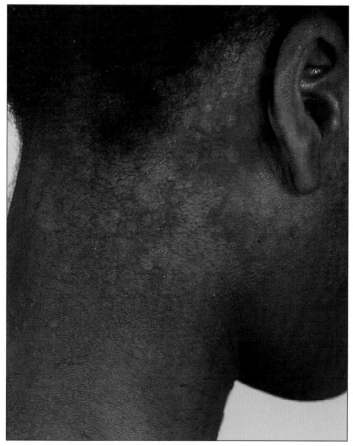

Figure 13 - Pityriasis versicolor.

Limited areas of pityriasis versicolor will respond to topical antifungal agents, such as *Canesten-HC* or *Daktarin*. Very extensive pityriasis versicolor can be treated with a three-day course of itraconazole (200 mg daily) but this will not prevent recurrence.

Candida albicans

Thrush affects mucosal surfaces as well as skin and is usually an opportunistic infection in patients who are immunocompromised, have diabetes or have been applying topical steroids. Candidal paronychia is particularly common in cleaners, housewives, etc., if they do not protect their hands from water, soap and detergents. Candidal paronychia can lead to secondary infection of the nail plate. This will need treatment with a topical imidazole such as *Trosyl* nail solution. In resistant cases, fluconazole orally can be used but terbinafine orally has little effect against *Candida* and griseofulvin has no effect.

Before starting patients on oral therapy for suspected fungal infection, it is very important that scrapings of the skin, clippings of nails or samples of hair are sent to a mycology department. Samples should be placed in dermopacks which can be obtained from the Microbiological Supply Company, PO Box 23 Toddington, Bedfordshire LU5 8DW. Samples can be sent locally or to:

Mycology Department
St John's Dermatology Centre
St Thomas' Hospital
London SE1 7EH.

HAIR LOSS

Hair loss from the scalp may either be patchy or diffuse. Patchy hair loss, other than that due to alopecia areata, probably merits referral to hospital. If diffuse hair loss is associated with a systemic illness or features of systemic lupus erythematosus (SLE) then hospital referral is again appropriate. Treatable causes of hair loss include thyroid dysfunction and iron deficiency anaemia, but these can be excluded with the appropriate investigations. Any subsequent hospital referral should be to the appropriate specialist.

If there is no evidence of any scalp disease, the remaining patients with diffuse alopecia will either have telogen effluvium, which will recover spontaneously, or constitutional alopecia which will not.

The only treatment for constitutional alopecia which has been shown to be effective is topical minoxidil (*Regaine*). It has been used in both men and women and it seems to work best in patients with less than five years of alopecia and in those with small bald areas at the vertex. It does not work well in patients with long-standing alopecia or in those in whom there is extensive hair loss. Treatment needs to be continued for at least six months, to establish whether hair regrowth is

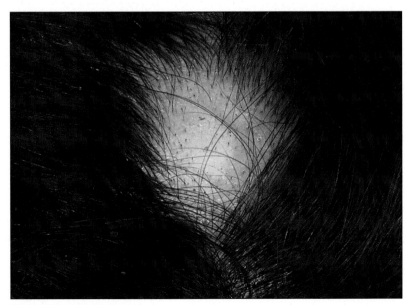

Figure 14 - Alopecia areata.

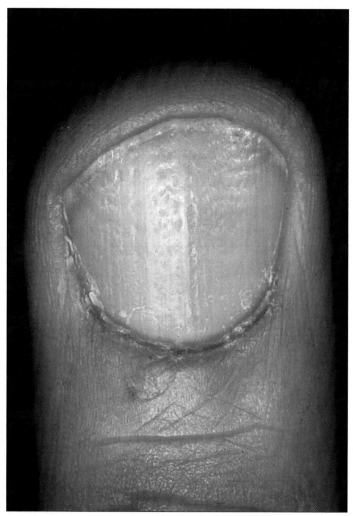

Figure 15 - Fine pitting of nails in alopecia areata.

occurring. The best studies indicate that only 30% of patients respond, but hair regrowth is very rarely complete. Furthermore, if hair regrowth does occur then therapy needs to be continued indefinitely as minoxidil has no permanent effect on hair growth. *Regaine* is expensive (£30 per month) but may become available over the counter.

HIRSUTIES

Excess facial hair in women is seldom the result of a virilising condition, unless there are associated features of virilisation, such as acne, irregular periods or male pattern hair loss. Pathological hirsuties is characterised by increase of muscle bulk, deepening of the voice, atrophy of the breasts, amenorrhoea and enlargement of the clitoris. In most females, facial hirsuties is genetically determined and often other women in the family are similarly affected. The problem can be dealt with by bleaching (with 1:10 hydrogen peroxide) or the use of depilatory cream. Many female patients with hirsuties reject advice to shave but are happy to accept the use of very fine emery paper, to remove fine hair on the face. Electrolysis can be used for terminal hairs but carries the risk of pigmentation or scarring, particularly in coloured patients. It is not routinely available on the NHS.

If the above measures are unsuccessful, anti-androgen therapy with a combination of ethinyloestradiol and cyproterone acetate is effective. However, patients with suspected virilisation or those requiring anti-androgen therapy should more appropriately be referred to an endocrinologist.

HYPERHIDROSIS

Patients with hyperhidrosis of the axillae or palms should be treated with aluminium chloride hexahydrate (*Anhydrol Forte* or *Driclor*). They should also be given appropriate instructions for the use of aluminium chloride hexahydrate:

1. Ensure that the area of skin is completely dry.

2. Do not shave armpits or use a depilatory cream within 24 hours of application.

3. Do not apply to broken or irritated skin.

4. Apply *Anhydrol Forte* or *Driclor* at night, prior to going to bed, and wash off thoroughly in the morning. Use for two nights in succession, followed by a rest period of two nights. Vary this according to how well you tolerate the application and your individual response. Many patients manage on one to two treatments per week, once the condition is under control. Transient irritation or redness may accompany use of *Anhydrol Forte*. Should this become excessive then stop the treatment and, if necessary, apply 1% hydrocortisone until the reaction has settled down.

Referral to hospital for hyperhidrosis should only be undertaken if the above measures have failed. Iontophoresis with glycopyrronium bromide in tap water can be used for hyperhidrosis of the palms and soles. Sympathectomy is considered only in the most severe and intractable cases.

NON-MELANOMA SKIN CANCERS AND PRECURSOR LESIONS

Under this title are included basal cell carcinomas and squamous cell carcinoma. Bowen's disease represents intra-epidermal carcinoma *in situ* and, like solar keratoses, should be considered as precursor lesions for squamous cell carcinoma. However, the chance of solar keratoses transforming into squamous cell carcinoma is low, probably 1:1,000 per year. If a patient only has one or two solar keratoses, the chance of developing a malignancy which requires treatment is small. If, however, the patient has 100 solar keratoses the chance of developing a squamous cell carcinoma is approximately 1:10 per year.

If you are unhappy about making the diagnosis of solar keratoses or Bowen's disease then the patient should be referred for an opinion. Bowen's disease can be treated by excision, cautery, cryotherapy or application of 5-fluorouracil (*Efudix*). The same principles apply to solar keratoses, but patients with multiple solar keratoses require *Efudix* in preference to the other treatment modalities. Some patients with solar keratoses do not require treatment or do not want treatment and can be kept under observation or instructed to return, should any of the lesions become nodular.

All patients with solar keratosis should be strongly advised to minimise their sun exposure, either by wearing a suitable hat or applying sunblock.

Topical *Retin-A* is effective in clearing solar keratoses if used over a sufficiently long period of time, and may

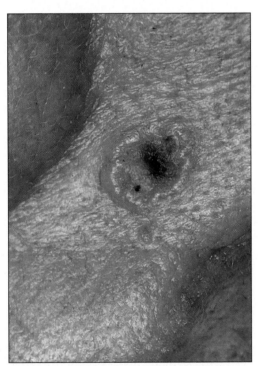

Figure 16 - Classic appearances of an early crusted basal cell carcinoma on the upper lip; note the pearly edge.

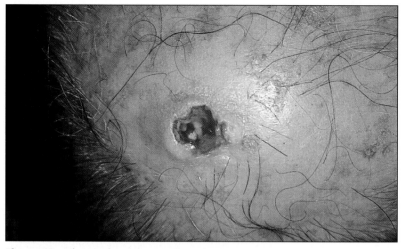

Figure 17 - Ulcerated squamous cell carcinoma on the scalp.

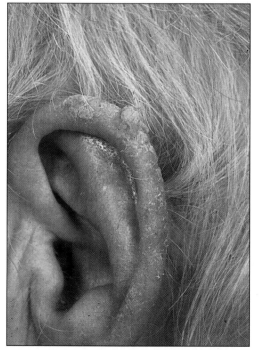

Figure 18 - Hyperkeratotic solar keratosis on ear.

prevent the occurrence of new lesions. However, it has to be applied on a daily basis for six months and lesions recur if treatment is discontinued. It is available as 0.025% and 0.05% cream.

ANY PATIENT REQUIRING A BIOPSY, OR IN WHOM EXCISION OF A SUSPECTED CANCER IS CONTEMPLAT-ED, REQUIRES REFERRAL TO HOSPITAL.

Dermatologists would much rather see lesions before they have been interfered with surgically. It compli-cates our task considerably if patients have already had biopsies or incomplete exci-sions of suspected skin cancers.

PIGMENTED
LESIONS

Malignant melanoma is the most rapidly increasing cancer at the present time. Over 3,000 new cases are reported annually in England and Wales, only slightly less than the number of new cervical cancer cases. Melanoma has a mortality of approximately 25% and prognosis is determined by the depth of invasion. Early diagnosis and referral is therefore essential and, for this reason, some hospitals have set up pigmented lesion clinics which are rapid-access clinics for patients with pigmented lesions. Other hospitals prefer to see patients urgently in the next available clinic.

However, many pigmented lesions are referred to hospital unnecessarily because of patient or parental anxiety. It is important to remember that moles develop in all people during childhood and puberty, and most young adults have 10 to 20 moles on their skin surface. It is extremely rare for melanoma to develop before puberty and such cases

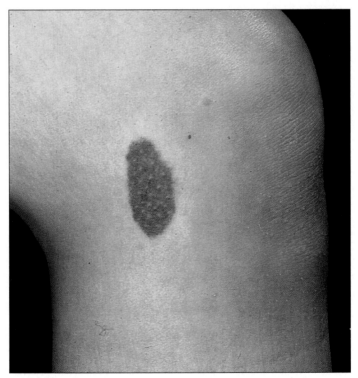

Figure 19 - A benign congenital melanocytic naevus.

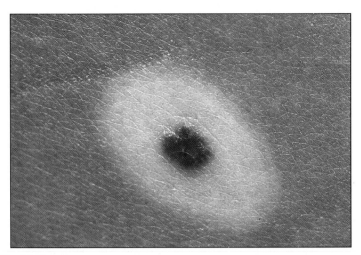

Figure 20 - A halo naevus.

usually arise in large congenital pigmented naevi. Just because a child develops a new mole, this does not require referral to hospital. Size is also a useful criteria. If, for example, a pigmented lesion is small enough that it can be covered by the blunt end of a pencil (4 mm) then melanoma is an unlikely diagnosis.

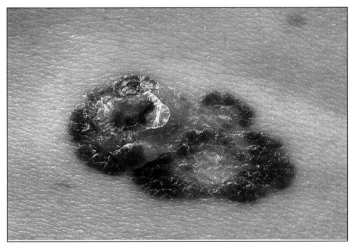

Figure 21 - A superficial spreading melanoma - note the irregularity of contour and pigmentation.

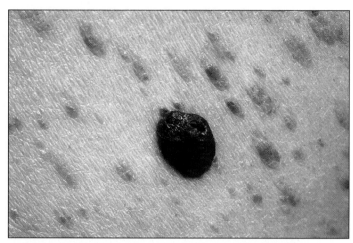

Figure 22 - Multiple pigmented seborrhoeic warts with a larger acanthotic pigmented seborrhoeic centrally. This can be distinguished from a melanoma by the presence of horn cysts within the surface of the lesion.

Another major cause for referral is pigmented lesions that are not of melanocytic origin. By far the commonest are pigmented seborrhoeic warts, which arise in older patients and can be recognised as pigmented lesions that are 'stuck onto the skin surface'. They may not

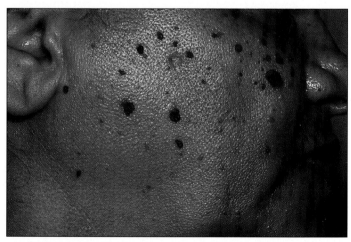

Figure 23 - Multiple pigmented seborrhoeic warts of the face (dermatosis papulosa nigrica).

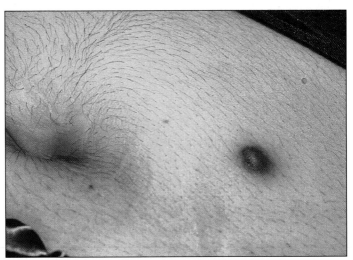

Figure 24 - A pigmented dermatofibroma below the elbow.

always be warty but most contain small keratin cysts which are visible macroscopically. Lesions are usually multiple; they vary considerably in size and in the degree of pigmentation; and because individual lesions can change size and shape and become inflamed, they are commonly referred as suspected melanomas.

A third source of confusion are dermatofibromas (also known as histiocytomas). These are firm, pigmented nodules, usually present on the legs. They often have a pigmented rim with a paler centre and, because of this variation in colour and also the tendency to itch, they are also referred as suspected melanomas.

If you are satisfied that the lesion is genuinely a melanocytic lesion, there are seven points which can help to identify an early malignant melanoma:

1. Is an existing mole enlarging, or is a new one growing? Moles do not usually change size after puberty.

2. Does it have a ragged or asymmetrical outline? Ordinary moles are smooth and regular.

3. Does it show irregular pigmentation? Ordinary moles may be dark brown or black but are usually uniform in colour.

Additional criteria include:

4. Size. Most normal moles can be covered by the blunt end of a pencil.

5. Is the mole inflamed?

6. Has it been bleeding, oozing or crusting?

7. Has there been any change in sensation? As a single feature this is probably the least useful, as many ordinary moles may itch if they become traumatised or if a hair follicle within the mole ruptures.

Again, we do not feel that any patient with a suspected melanoma should have surgery prior to referral. Obviously, if a mole is being removed for cosmetic reasons, that is a matter for the patient and the GP. Equally, if there is any doubt about diagnosis, patients can be seen urgently.

PROTECTION FROM SUNLIGHT

Patients with fair skin, a history of sunburn, photo-dermatoses, such as polymorphic light eruption, solar keratoses and particularly those with a history of melanoma or non-melanoma skin cancer, require sun protection. Sunblocks either consist of chemicals which absorb ultraviolet rays or physical sunblocks which reflect ultraviolet light. However, they are expensive, there is often a problem with compliance and clothing is a more effective method of screening out ultraviolet light than creams or ointments. Remember that the relationship between skin cancer risk and ultraviolet dose is not linear but exponential. This means that once patients have accumulated a certain ultraviolet dose, each further increment in dose carries with it a disproportionate increase in skin cancer risk. It is therefore not logical for patients to say, "Well, there is no point in protecting my skin now, as all the damage has been done previously". There is always every reason for protecting the skin of patients who are at risk of developing skin cancer.

The effectiveness of sunblocks is indicated by the sun protection factor (SPF) number, which usually ranges from 4 to 30. If a sunblock has an SPF of 10, this means that the patient can spend 10 hours in the sun and will receive the same amount of ultraviolet light to the skin as if they were unprotected for one hour.

However, the SPF is calculated by measuring erythema in volunteer subjects and reflects the amount of UVB protection offered by the sunblock. Whilst there is a very good correlation between UV-induced erythema and the production of skin cancer in animal models, it is not true to say that only UVB is carcinogenic. Longer wavelength ultraviolet light, UVA, may be less potent at producing erythema or cancer but exposure to UVA in the general population is much higher than for UVB and continues throughout the year. Consequently, many sunblock manufacturers are now including an assessment of UVA protection in their sunblocks, as well as the SPF. Sunblocks which can be prescribed for patients with photosensitive eruptions or vitiligo are listed in the *British National Formulary*. All these have an SPF of 15 or greater, and most offer UVA as well as UVB protection. *Uvistat* ultrablock cream, for example, offers good UVA and UVB protection with an SPF of 30.

Sunscreens should be used in the following way:

1. Apply before breakfast every day from April to September inclusive.

2. On days when the sun is out, apply at lunchtime as well.

3. Use sunblock under other skin creams or make-up.

4. Re-apply after swimming or use a waterproof sunblock.

5. Use on all light-exposed areas; that is, face, hands, V of neck and don't forget the ears.

PIGMENTATION

One of the most distressing sequelae of almost any inflammatory skin disease is pigmentary changes in the skin which may either be loss of pigment (hypopigmentation) or hyperpigmentation. However, this type of post-inflammatory pigmentation is not amenable to treatment, other than treatment for the underlying disease. It can, of course, be dealt with by cosmetic camouflage.

Vitiligo

Areas of pigment loss not preceded by any inflammatory skin disease are usually due to vitiligo. This is regarded as an autoimmune disorder and may be associated with other autoimmune diseases, such as alopecia areata, pernicious anaemia or autoimmune thyroid disease. Appropriate investigations can be carried out, not to confirm the diagnosis of vitiligo but to exclude associated diseases which can be treated.

Treatment for vitiligo is generally unsatisfactory.

1. New areas of pigment loss can be treated by a very potent topical steroid. Daily treatment for one month only is usually recommended.

2. For patients with vitiligo on the face, cosmetic camouflage can transform their lives. Expert cosmetic advice can be obtained from the Red Cross or privately from a qualified beautician. *Dermablend* cosmetic products are available on prescription.

3. Psoralen plus ultraviolet A (PUVA) treatment has been used in patients with extensive vitiligo. However, it is less effective in patients with long-standing vitiligo and in those with vitiligo at acral sites. Treatment needs to be continued for at least six months and the final cosmetic result is not always satisfactory.

4. It should be remembered that patients with vitiligo cannot pigment as a result of sun exposure and require advice about sunblocks and sun avoidance.

Chloasma

Pregnant women and women taking the oral contraceptive may develop facial pigmentation due to increased production of melanin

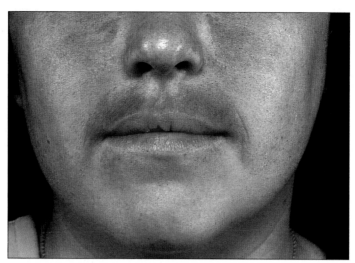

Figure 25 - Chloasma; note bilateral symmetrical pigmentation of cheeks and upper lip.

within the epidermis. This is aggravated by sun exposure and such patients should use sunblocks and practise sun avoidance. Depigmenting agents such as 5% hydroquinone in 1% hydrocortisone cream can be used for chloasma but not during pregnancy. Such women require advice on alternative methods of contraception.

Facial pigmentation may also be seen in individuals who have neither been pregnant nor taken the contraceptive pill. Such patients may have been exposed to photosensitising chemicals, e.g. plant extracts containing psoralens which are used in perfumes and cosmetics. Such patients should be advised to use non-perfumed soap, e.g. *Simple* soap, and to use hypoallergenic make-up (*RoC* or *Almay*). Equally, female patients may have developed an allergic contact dermatitis to their cosmetics and this requires referral for patch testing.

Depigmenting creams are ineffective if melanin is located in the dermis; they are therefore ineffective in patients with eczema, lichen planus, etc. who have post-inflammatory hyperpigmentation. In fact, they may aggravate the problem by depigmenting the surrounding normal skin and highlighting the abnormally pigmented skin.

PSORIASIS

Psoriasis affects approximately 2% of the population. Like eczema, it is a chronic inflammatory skin condition but is more resistant than eczema to topical steroids; many patients with psoriasis get referred to hospital only because the patient insists on a specialist opinion. However, unless a patient requires daily outpatient therapy, phototherapy with UVB and PUVA, or cytotoxic therapy with methotrexate or cyclosporin, there is no need for patients with stable plaque psoriasis to be followed up in a hospital department. Topical therapies for psoriasis are well standardised and all GPs should be familiar with them.

1. Use a soap substitute such as aqueous cream and a liquid tar preparation such as *Polytar* emollient or *Balneum with Tar* in the bath.

2. Apply a moisturiser after bathing. For particularly scaly psoriasis 50/50 mixture is the most effective (contains 50% white soft paraffin:50% liquid paraffin).

3. A mild or moderate topical steroid is adequate for many patients with psoriasis. In children, hydrocortisone can be combined with tar in products such as *Tarcortin* and *Alphosyl HC*. More potent steroids can be used in adults, for

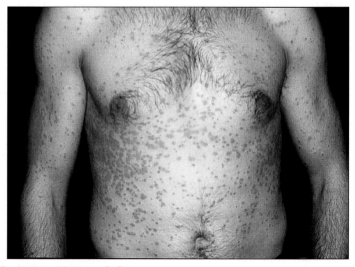

Figure 26 - Acute guttate psoriasis.

example 25% *Betnovate* with 5% LPC, but some patients find the tar content cosmetically unacceptable. A potent steroid combined with a keratolytic agent (e.g. *Diprosalic*) can be useful in hyperkeratotic areas

.4.For those patients who are resistant to steroids or dislike using them, calcipotriol (e.g. *Dovonex*) is a suitable alternative. Cosmetically it is more acceptable than alternatives such as coal tar or dithranol but it is mildly irritant, should not be used on the face and should be used with care at flexural sites. Initially, treatment should be given twice daily for four to six weeks and continued if improvement occurs. Unless very extensive areas of psoriasis are being treated, hypercalcaemia is not usually a problem. If irritation occurs, *Dovonex* can be used in conjunction with a topical steroid.

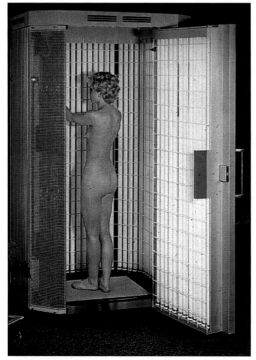

Figure 27 - A stand-up PUVA machine with the door open.

Coal tar and dithranol

In hospital, either in the outpatient day treatment centre or as an inpatient, UVB is often combined with increasing concentrations of coal tar applied topically (Goeckerman regime) or increasing concentrations of dithranol applied topically (Ingram's regime). Coal tar is not very suitable for use in the home as it is messy and smelly and most patients stop using it. However, short-contact dithranol treatment can be used in the home, provided appropriate instructions are given, as follows:

1. Apply dithranol to all scaly patches of psoriasis (use rubber

gloves). Start with the lowest concentration (0.25%), do not treat the face and avoid any sore areas or any flexural areas such as the armpit or groin, where skin surfaces rub together. Try to ensure that the paste does not spread onto the normal skin around the patch of psoriasis. Leave on for 15 minutes.

2. At the end of this time, remove the application using Arachis oil followed by a bath or a shower.

3. Increase the length of application by 15 minutes every third day, to a maximum of one hour. If a period of one hour's treatment has been reached and the psoriasis is not responding then go on to the higher concentration of dithranol (0.5%, 1%, 2% can be used). Remember, when you increase the concentration, go back to the original 15 minutes and then build up the time as before

Cautions:

1. Dithranol will do harm to normal skin. If you get it on your fingers, wash it off. Avoid contact with the eyes.

2. Dithranol stains clothing and bedding. Use old clothes such as an old pair of pyjamas or a dressing gown whilst the dithranol is on your skin.

3. Keep the ointment out of reach of children.

4. If the treated area becomes painful, stop treatment for two days, apply emulsifying ointment or a topical steroid and then resume treatment but cut down the time of treatment by half an hour and build up again as before.

Finally, explain to patients that their treatment is successful when the psoriasis has stopped scaling and the skin becomes smooth. The brown staining associated with dithranol treatment will fade in the course of time.

Psoriasis of the scalp

The scalp is commonly affected by psoriasis, either alone or in combination with psoriasis elsewhere. The other common condition affecting the scalp is seborrhoeic eczema, and these can be quite difficult to

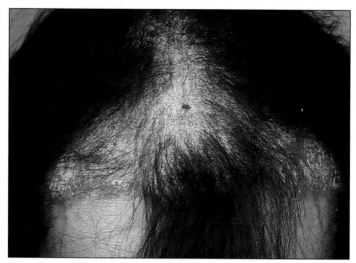

Figure 28 - Psoriasis involving the scalp; note the geographical border and involvement of non-hair bearing skin.

distinguish if the scalp alone is affected. However, from the point of view of treatment this is not so critical, as the following treatment is common to both conditions:

- Apply *Ung Cocois Co* by rubbing into the scalp before going to bed and leave on overnight. *Cocois* is an alternative product which is available commercially. *Ung Cocois Co* is a brown ointment and users are advised to wear a scarf or handkerchief to protect the sheets and pillow cases.

- In the morning, wash out the *Ung Cocois Co* with a suitable medicated shampoo (*Polytar, Genisol, Alphosyl* etc.). If scaling or itching persists during the day a potent steroid application can be used (e.g. *Synlar Gel, Betnovate* or *Locoid* scalp application, *Elocon Lotion,* etc).

For patients with psoriasis of the scalp, *Dovonex* scalp application is now available but trials indicate that it is no more effective than *Betnovate* scalp application. However, it may be more effective in individual patients or preferred by other patients.

Patients require referral to hospital if their psoriasis is resistant to the above treatments. It is important, however, not to raise unrealistic expectations in patients with psoriasis. The tendency to develop psoriasis is life-long and treatment will control, not cure, the condition. Remember that some drugs can exacerbate psoriasis (e.g. lithium) and some drugs can produce a psoriasiform eruption, particularly methyldopa and beta-blockers. In this situation, hospital referral is appropriate. It is also appropriate for patients with acute guttate psoriasis where UVB therapy alone is often effective.

For further advice, patients can contact:

The Psoriasis Association
7 Milton Street
Northampton NN2 7JF.
Tel: 01604 711129
Fax: 01604 711129

Table 3 Management of psoriasis

		Scalp
Mild psoriasis	• Bath emollients (tar based) • Moisturiser after bath • Tar/steroid mixture topically (e.g. *Tarcortin*; *Alphosyl HC* b.d.) **or** *Dovonex* ung. b.d.	• Tar-based shampoo • Potent topical steroid (e.g. *Synalar Gel* o.d.) **or** *Dovonex* scalp application
Moderate psoriasis	As above plus: • Soap substitute • Moderately potent steroid ± 5% LPC **or** dithranol - short contact (0.25 - 2%)	• Add cocois co. to scalp overnight • Dithranol pommade
Severe psoriasis	As above Refer to hospital for: • Outpatient/inpatient therapy with crude coal tar (CCT) or dithranol in Lassar's paste, applied in increasing concentrations under stockingette. Medium contact (four to six hours) or long contact (10 - 12 hours). Above usually combined with phototherapy (UVB x 3 weekly) **or** PUVA x 2 weekly ± retinoids (*Neotigason*) **or** cytotoxic therapy: methotrexate, cyclosporin-A, etc.	

SCABIES

In general, use gamma benzene hexachloride (*Quellada*) with a week between each application or benzyl benzoate on two successive days. Treatments for scabies are usually irritant, particularly benzyl benzoate, so if a child has eczema and is given a therapeutic trial of antiscabetic treatment, the eczema will usually deteriorate.

In infants and very young children malathion or possibly *Eurax* is preferable, because of the small and rather theoretical risk of significant absorption and cerebral damage from gamma benzene hexachloride. Ten per cent sulphur ointment is the treatment of choice for pregnant women.

If a patient continues to itch after properly-applied treatment, then prescribe a soothing cream such as calamine or a mild steroid ointment such as 1% hydrocortisone.

Patients with scabies often continue to itch for seven to 10 days after treatment, even though all the mites have been killed, so there is no point in continuing with antiscabetic therapy. More important is to ensure that all contacts in the household are treated simultaneously.

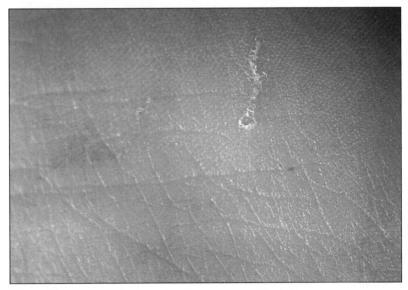

Figure 29 - Close-up of a typical scabies burrow on the palm.

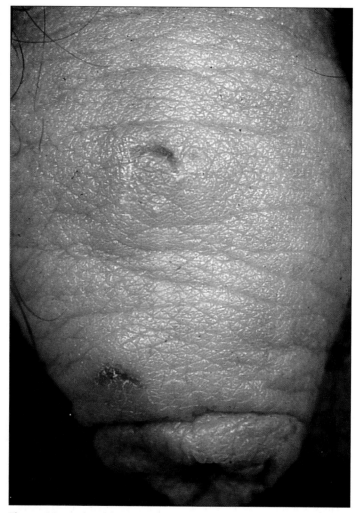

Figure 30 - Scabetic lesions on the penis.

After treatment, all members of the household should have a complete change of towels, sheets, pillow cases and underclothes. Other garments can be washed or ironed or left unworn for a week, as the mite does not survive off the human host for more than a day or so.

ULCERS

The most appropriate form of management for chronic venous ulceration in elderly patients is by appropriately-trained nurses in the community, and community-based ulcer clinics have now been established in many areas of London. However, the most important initial step is to establish whether ulcers are of venous origin, arterial origin or a mixture of both, or due to some other cause, such as a haemoglobinopathy (e.g. sickle-cell disease). Compression bandaging is clearly inappropriate in patients who have predominantly arterial ulceration and, where doubt exists, referral to a vascular clinic is appropriate.

With the establishment of community ulcer clinics, dermatology departments have become less involved with the long-term management of venous ulceration. However, referrals are still appropriate if the surrounding skin becomes inflamed. There are four basic reasons for this:

1. Secondary infection (cellulitis)

2. Acute or chronic lipodermatosclerosis

3. Varicose eczema

4. Allergic contact dermatitis to the topically-applied medicaments. In this situation, patch testing is appropriate.

As a general rule, venous ulcers will heal if the patient rests with the legs elevated and the ulcer is cleaned on a regular basis. Although expensive dressings are heavily promoted by drug companies, there is no evidence that any dressing accelerates the rate at which ulcers heal naturally. Because patients are reluctant to stay in bed, compression bandaging is essential when patients are ambulant. Four-layer compression bandaging represents a major advance in ulcer care and all nurses who are looking after patients with ulcers should be familiar with its use and application.

Ulcers which become infected should be soaked daily, either with phenoxyethanol, if *Pseudomonas* is cultured, or with potassium permanganate 1:8,000. Oral antibiotics have little part to play in the management of chronic venous ulceration unless there is an associated cellulitis or folliculitis.

URTICARIA

Most patients with urticaria should be managed in the GP surgery. It is important to ask relevant questions to rule out physical causes of urticaria, such as cholinergic urticaria, cold urticaria, aquagenic urticaria and dermographism.

Acute episodes of urticaria may have an obvious cause; either a drug or foods which are well known to produce acute urticarial reactions (shellfish, fruits, nuts, etc.). Persistent episodes of urticaria which last more than three months are defined as chronic urticaria and here an allergic cause is seldom found.

Routine investigations should be carried out to exclude any associated diseases and these should include thyroid function tests, routine biochemistry, full blood count and erythrocyte sedimentation rate (ESR). Patients with urticaria and a high ESR need referral for exclusion of autoimmune disease and urticarial vasculitis.

Patients with chronic urticaria do not require skin testing either with prick tests or patch tests. The vast majority of patients with chronic urticaria remit spontaneously within six months. About 40% of patients find that their urticaria is aggravated by exposure to salicylates, so tell all patients to avoid all aspirin-containing drugs. Paracetamol should be used as an alternative analgesic.

If chronic urticaria persists beyond six months, dietary manipulation can be tried in co-operation with a dietitian. Diets free of salicylates, azodyes and preservatives are effective in a minority of patients, but there is no point in continuing if there is no response after four weeks.

Antihistamines

Antihistamines are still the mainstay of treatment for chronic urticaria. Terfenadine (*Triludan*) and astemizole (*Hismanal*) are less sedating than older drugs but there have been concerns about dysrhythmias with high doses. They should be avoided in patients with a history of dysrhythmia or patients taking erythromycin or other macrolides.

Alternative antihistamines, which only need to be taken once daily, include loratadine (*Clarityn* 10 mg daily) and cetirizine (*Zirtek* 10 mg daily). Both products are becoming increasingly popular because of their lack of significant cardiovascular effects as well as lack of sedation. If these are ineffective, then the more old-fashioned sedating antihistamines can still be very effective (e.g. *Piriton*, *Dimotane Plus* or *Atarax*).

VIRUSES
AND WARTS

Two of the commonest viral infections seen in children are molluscum contagiosum and viral warts due to the human papilloma virus (HPV).

Molluscum contagiosum

Many dermatologists are reluctant to treat molluscum contagiosum in small children as there is no treatment that is painless. Older children may tolerate cryotherapy, application of liquidised phenol or puncturing the lesion with a needle or a sharpened orange stick. At home, the parent can be taught to squeeze the lesions between the thumb nails after soaking in the bath.

Molluscum contagiosum has a limited duration of six months to one year and will therefore remit spontaneously, even if no treatment is given. There is, of course, a risk of transmission to other children as the condition is contagious, but there is no justification for keeping children who have molluscum contagiosum off school.

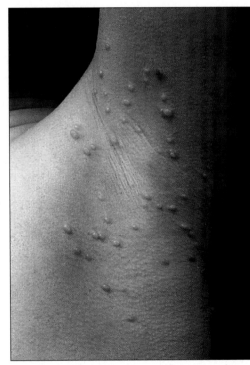

Figure 31 - Multiple lesions of molluscum contagiosum.

Viral warts

Patients with small plane warts require treatment with a suitable wart remedy such as *Salactol* but this should not be applied to the face. Otherwise, viral warts can be left alone, treated with topical wart remedies or treated with cryotherapy. Since spontaneous resolution in warts is extremely common, cryotherapy should be delayed wherever possible, to give the lesions a chance to remit. Liquid nitrogen is a painful treatment and children do not tolerate it well.

As a general rule, children under five years are never treated, and children under 10 years rarely. There is no point in referring patients with warts for laser treatment as this is not generally available and there is no good evidence that it is more effective than other methods of destroying warts.

Although it is recommended that children with genital warts should be referred to the paediatric department for exclusion of sexual abuse, it is important to recognise that hand warts can be readily transmitted to the anogenital area through quite normal activities. Adults with genital warts should be referred to the genitourinary clinic as contact tracing is important.

Cryotherapy in general practice

A wide variety of benign skin lesions can be treated with cryotherapy,

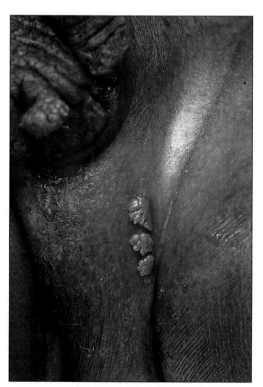

apart from viral warts. In particular, seborrhoeic warts and skin tags. However, a more effective treatment for skin tags is to remove them under local anaesthetic, either by snipping them off with scissors or by cutting them with a cautery. Large seborrhoeic warts can easily be removed by curettage under local anaesthetic with diathermy cauterisation of the base. Liquid nitrogen can be made available through the hospital pharmacy for those practices who wish to avail themselves of it. GPs can also arrange for supplies to be delivered directly by the British Oxygen Company.

Figure 32 - Filiform genital warts in the crural area.